How To Get Rid Of A Yeast Infection

330 Great Tips To Prevent And Cure Candida Yeast Infection

ADAM COLTON

Published by BizMove
www.bizmove.com

ISBN: 1979001057
ISBN- 978-1979001052

Table of Contents

1. Yeast Infection Fact Sheet

Vaginal yeast infection is an infection of the vagina. It is most commonly due to the fungus *Candida albicans.*

Causes

Most women have a vaginal yeast infection at some time. *Candida albicans* is a common type of fungus. It is often found in small amounts in the vagina, mouth, digestive tract, and on the skin. Most of the time, it does not cause infection or symptoms.

Candida and the many other germs that normally live in the vagina keep each other in balance. However, sometimes the number of *Candida* increases, leading to a yeast infection.

This can happen if:

- You are taking antibiotics used to treat another infection. Antibiotics change the normal balance between germs in the vagina.
- You are pregnant
- You are obese
- You have diabetes

A yeast infection is not spread through sexual contact. However, some men will develop symptoms such as itching and a rash on the penis after having sexual contact with an infected partner.

Having many vaginal yeast infections may be a sign of other health problems. Other vaginal infections and discharges can be mistaken for a vaginal yeast infection.

Symptoms

Symptoms include:

- Abnormal vaginal discharge. Discharge can range from slightly watery, white discharge to thick, white, and chunky (like cottage cheese).
- Itching and burning of the vagina and labia
- Pain with intercourse
- Painful urination
- Redness and swelling of the skin just outside of the vagina (vulva)

Exams and Tests

You will have a pelvic exam. It may show:

- Swelling and redness of the skin of the vulva, in the vagina, and on the cervix
- Dry, white spots on the vaginal wall
- Cracks in the skin of the vulva.

A small amount of the vaginal discharge is examined using a microscope. This is called a wet mount and KOH test.

Sometimes, a culture is taken when the infection does not get better with treatment or comes back many times.

Your health care provider may order other tests to rule out other causes of your symptoms.

Treatment

Medicines to treat vaginal yeast infections are available as creams, ointments, vaginal tablets or suppositories and oral tablets. Most can be bought without needing to see your provider.

Treating yourself at home is probably OK if:

- Your symptoms are mild and you do not have pelvic pain or a fever
- This is not your first yeast infection and you have not had many yeast infections in the past
- You are not pregnant
- You are not worried about other sexually transmitted infections from recent sexual contact

Medicines you can buy yourself to treat a vaginal yeast infection are:

- Miconazole
- Clotrimazole
- Tioconazole
- Butoconazole

When using these medicines:

- Read the packages carefully and use them as directed.
- You will need to take the medicine for 1 to 7 days, depending on which medicine you buy. (If you do not get repeated infections, a 1-day medicine might work for you.)
- Do not stop using these medicines early because your symptoms are better.

You doctor can also prescribe a pill that you only take by mouth once.

If your symptoms are worse or you get vaginal yeast infections often, you may need:

- Medicine for up to 14 days
- Clotrimazole vaginal suppository or fluconazole pill every week to prevent new infections

To help prevent and treat vaginal discharge:

- Keep your genital area clean and dry. Avoid soap and rinse with water only. Sitting in a warm, but not hot, bath may help your symptoms.

- Avoid douching. Although many women feel cleaner if they douche after their period or intercourse, it may worsen vaginal discharge. Douching removes healthy bacteria lining the vagina that protect against infection.
- Eat yogurt with live cultures or take *Lactobacillus acidophilus* tablets when you are on antibiotics. This may help to prevent a yeast infection.
- Use condoms to avoid catching or spreading other infections.
- Avoid using feminine hygiene sprays, fragrances, or powders in the genital area.
- Avoid wearing tight-fitting pants or shorts, which may cause irritation.
- Wear cotton underwear or cotton-crotch pantyhose. Avoid underwear made of silk or nylon, because they can increase sweating in the genital area, which leads to growth of more yeast.
- Keep your blood sugar level under good control if you have diabetes.
- Avoid wearing wet bathing suits or exercise clothing for long periods of time. Wash sweaty or wet clothes after each use.

Outlook (Prognosis)

Most of the time, symptoms go away completely with proper treatment.

Possible Complications

A lot of scratching may cause the skin to crack, making you more likely to get a skin infection.

Repeat infections that occur right after treatment, or a yeast infection that does not respond well to treatment, may be an early sign of diabetes or rarely, HIV.

When to Contact a Medical Professional

Call your provider if:

- This is the first time that you have had symptoms of a vaginal yeast infection.
- You are not sure if you have a yeast infection.
- Your symptoms don't go away after using over-the-counter medicines.
- Your symptoms get worse.
- You develop other symptoms.
- You may have been exposed to an STD.

2. 330 Great Tips To Prevent And Cure Candida Yeast Infection

The human body is an amazing thing, but sometimes it just doesn't work as well as we want it to. If you are prone to yeast infections, or simply looking for ways to avoid them, read the following tips. It will teach you ways of preventing yeast infections and the best treatment, should you happen to get one.

1. One of the things that you will want to make sure of during the day is to wear all natural clothing. Try to stick predominantly to cotton and silk as these materials can help prevent moisture on your body, versus other materials such as nylon, which can yield more moisture.

2. The best way to prevent yeast infections is to dress properly. Cotton and silk are natural fibers that absorb moisture and will help keep the area dry. Nylon and other man made fabrics will not absorb moisture as well, and you will increase the likelihood of getting a yeast infection.

3. In order to prevent yeast infections, especially in women, limit the amount of time you spend in the heat. This means to limit time you spend bathing in hot water. Yeast organisms love hot and moist areas; therefore they thrive. Furthermore, remember to avoid wearing any tight clothing that can stop proper air circulation in the crotch area.

4. Avoid anything scented near the genital area. Anything from sprays to soaps to scented pads can cause a yeast infection. This is particularly crucial for things that come in direct contact with this area like pads and tampons because that can cause a lot of irritation. Avoid using colored toilet paper, too.

5. If you suffer from a yeast infection, or would just like to take preventative measures, make sure that you drink plenty of water. Your water intake should be about 10 to 12 glasses of water each day. By taking the effort to drink enough water, you are flushing toxins and bacteria out of your system.

6. Douching is a common cause of yeast infections. Douching is supposed to help clean your body, but it can actually bring about a yeast infection. Douching upsets the natural balance of bacteria in your vagina. When your vagina is unbalanced, you are more likely to get an infection.

7. While less common that vaginal ones, oral yeast infections do happen. Always contact your doctor if you think you might have an infection. Rinsing the mouth with a warm saltwater solution, or drinking liquids that are cool, can help to minimize discomfort.

8. If you have a yeast infection, try using an over-the-counter antifungal cream. You can find these at your local grocery store or drug store. They are available under different names like Vagisil and Monistat. Apply the cream as directed to the affected area to help soothe and treat the symptoms of yeast infection.

9. Always opt for a quick shower instead of a long hot bath, if you are at all prone to developing yeast infections. Yeast thrives in hot, moist environments and despite how soothing a soak in the tub can be, it will also be an engraved invitation to another yeast infection.

10. You can prevent yeast infections by improving your hygiene. Wash your vagina with a special soap: choose a product with a neutral PH if possible and douche once a week. Use mouthwash and floss to get rid of the bacteria present in your mouth. Use a clean towel to dry after showering.

11.   Your dietary intake can be an important factor in the battle against yeast infections! Studies show that eating yogurt with active cultures can help lower the amount of yeast in the body, thereby reducing the number of yeast infections you may get. Also, consider lowering the amount of sugar you consume, as another benefit to yeast reduction.

12.   While many people may believe that douching is a good way to prevent the onset of yeast infections this is actually not the case. Douching destroys both harmful as well as helpful bacteria that can help prevent yeast infections from occurring. Do yourself a favor and stay away from douching.

13.   Try using tea tree oil. Tea tree oil can sometimes offer you instant relief from your yeast infection. Only use a tiny amount. Be careful when applying it. Some people do find that it burns. It would be a good idea to speak to a doctor before trying this yourself.

14.   A few simple changes to your daily dieting habits are an easy solution for preventing harmful yeast infections. It has been shown that foods with sugar promote yeast, while foods like yogurt have natural cultures that keep yeast away.

15.   Apple cider vinegar is great to help cure and relieve the symptoms of a yeast infection. While you can put it directly on the vagina, it will burn like crazy. Instead, add a cup or so to a hot bath. It will help kill the yeast and relieve the itching.

16.   Do not use anti-fungal medications in or around the vagina that are intended for treating other kinds of yeast. Medications meant for athlete's foot or nail fungus may not be effective against vaginal yeast. They can also be too strong or irritating for delicate skin or internal use. Stick to the medications formulated for use around the genitals.

17.   Those that suffer from diabetes should take extra care to keep their blood sugar levels under control if they wish to prevent a yeast infection from occurring. If your blood sugar is too high, or too low you have a much greater risk of developing a yeast infection than someone with normal blood sugar.

18.   A good tip to remember if you don't want to end up getting a yeast infection is to be careful about the medications you're currently using. Research has shown that if you've recently been using antibiotics or oral steroids you might be at more of a risk for getting a yeast infection.

19.   When you've finished an activity that causes you to expend a lot of your energy, put on new clothes. This will make you less prone to getting a yeast infection.

20.   Be aware of the impact of birth control pills. Not only do they help prevent pregnancy, but birth control pills usually contain estrogen as well. Taking estrogen in this way can cause fluctuations in the vagina's natural balance. When this occurs, the environment for yeast growth can be created. If infections are common for you, consult with your physician about options that can help.

21.   Avoid wearing tight, skinny jeans. While these types of jeans are cute and popular in the fashion arena, they make it more difficult for air to get to the crotch region, and this can cause yeast infections. It's better to wear looser pants or even a skirt whenever possible.

22.   If you suffer from yeast infections, some changes in your diet may be helpful in keeping them at bay. Try eating yogurt with live cultures that combat yeast. Also, try to eliminate as much sugar as possible from your diet, as sugar has been shown to help yeast to grow.

23.   If you have a yeast infection, do not try to douche. A douche might provide temporary relief from itching, but it can disturb the natural flora balance and make your yeast infection more severe. Make sure to discuss any douche you might want to use with your physician before giving it a try.

24.   Purchase specialized soap designed for the genital area and use only this for washing these parts. There are many great products on the market. They are formulated to keep the balance of a woman's body in check and will keep the area from becoming dry or unbalanced. Selecting them rather than typical soaps is a good way to prevent yeast infections.

25.   Although they are not seen nearly as much as vaginal yeast infections, the oral cavity is susceptible to yeast infection as well. If this happens, make sure you see your doctor as soon as possible. Warm saltwater is effective in this situation, as is the consumption of cool liquids.

26.   Curing a yeast infection does not have to take a long time. There are several very effective one day treatments available. These can be purchased over the counter at your local pharmacy or supermarket. Give one a try and see if it offers the relief you need from that troublesome infection.

27.   If you suffer from reoccurring yeast infections, visit your doctor. While there are many very effective over the counter treatments, a reoccurring infection warrants a doctor's visit. A doctor can help you to determine the underlying cause and keep those infections from coming back. They also might be able to offer some stronger medications to cure your infection faster.

28.   Try eating more garlic. Adding a little more garlic to your diet can do wonders if you suffer from yeast infections. Studies have found that garlic has the ability to kill off yeast. This can be used to get rid of yeast infections and may prevent them from reoccurring in the future.

29.   To cut down on your chances or impact from a yeast infection, stay thoroughly hydrated. The often you urinate, the more likely you are to flush excess sugars out of your system. This drastically cuts down on both your chances of a yeast infection and the lifespan of any current ones.

30.   Know the differences between yeast infections and bacterial infections. A yeast infection causes itching, burning, redness and discharge that looks like cottage cheese. Bacterial infections cause foul smells, itching, irritation and discharge that may

appear yellowish or greenish in color. If you aren't sure which type you have, seek medical attention before attempting treatment.

31.   Keep your immune system strong with plenty of sleep and proper nutrition. A lowered immune system can lead to an increase in all kinds of infections, including yeast growth. If you have diabetes or are undergoing chemotherapy, your immune system is lowered, and you may be more prone to yeast infections.

32.   One thing you can do to beat yeast infections is to make a few dietary changes. Sugars are shown to promote yeast infections and sugar-free yogurt can actually help rid you of one.

33.   Consume lots of liquids! Eight daily glasses is a common recommendation for the average adult, but you should drink plenty more during a yeast infection. You urinate much more frequently when you drink a lot of water throughout the day. Urinating naturally flushes out natural sugars that yeast feeds on.

34.   Be mindful of the fact that yeast is quite commonly found in your intestinal system. When you use the restroom, make sure to wipe from front first to the back. This should prevent any yeast

from making it into the vaginal area, and will cut down dramatically on your chances of an infection.

35.   Eat lots and lots of garlic. Garlic has many benefits, including anti-fungal properties. The anti-fungal properties of garlic can help to prevent and treat yeast infections. However, garlic can thin your blood, so if you are taking any blood thinning medications, consult with your general practitioner before upping your garlic intake.

36.   Boric acid suppositories have been proven effective in fighting yeast infections. Boric acid destroys harmful micro organisms, including yeast. When used in suppository form, it has been scientifically proven to provide a high level of relief. A pregnant Woman should not use this method, and a doctor should be consulted if use will be long term.

37.   Cinnamon is a wonderful herb that can help reduce the effects of infection if you happen to catch a yeast infection. You can sprinkle a little amount of cinnamon on many different things, whether you are using it on a meal or dessert to help reduce the chances of infection in your body.

38.   If you spend time in a pool or sauna, always remove your damp clothing when done. Avoid

wearing any wet clothing as it can promote yeast growth. Make sure you are completely dry once the wet clothes are removed, and then go ahead and put on dry clothes.

39.   If you have a yeast infection, try to reduce the hot and spicy foods that you eat during your meals and snacks. These types of foods can aggravate the infections that you have any make you feel very uncomfortable. Eat moderate foods if you want to feel comfortable with a yeast infection.

40.   For a natural way to fight a mild yeast infection, turn to your pantry for a clove of garlic. You can create a suppository with the garlic by nicking it with a knife and inserting it into the vagina overnight. If you are worried about retrieving it, use a needle to pull a piece of string through the clove. If you experience any irritation, remove the clove promptly.

41.   Make sure you dry yourself very thoroughly after bathing and showering to prevent yeast infections. Yeast thrive in moist environments, including folds of skin found almost anywhere on the body. Gently pat the skin dry with an absorbent towel, and then apply body powder to these areas to absorb even more moisture.

42.   If you try to treat your yeast infection at home, see a doctor after a week if it has not cleared up. There are many over-the-counter treatments for yeast infections these days, as well as many home remedies you can try. However, after a week you must realize that you need medical attention so that the infection does not worsen.

43.   Did you know that the bacteria in plain yogurt can help fight a yeast infection? It is true, but it has to be unsweetened yogurt. Yeast feeds on sugar and yogurt will not be helpful if it contains sugar. You can even use it as a topical treatment by dipping a tampon in yogurt.

44.   Garlic is a great natural remedy, and it has proven effective in fighting yeast infections. Create a garlic tampon by tying string to a couple of cloves and inserting it into the vagina. Leave it in for a couple of hours, and relief will typically come. The antifungal properties of the garlic have a healing effect and can effectively combat troublesome yeast.

45.   An important tip for preventing the occurrence of yeast infections is to avoid lingering in a wet bathing suit for a prolonged period of time. By getting out of wet swimsuits as soon as possible after swimming, you have the power to deprive

yeast of the warm, damp environment in which they thrive.

46.   Many women think that douching will keep the vaginal area clean and less susceptible to yeast infection. However, frequent douching can actually destroy the good bacteria that live in the vagina, leaving you more likely to get a yeast infection. Regular bathing with a gentle cleanser and thorough drying are enough to keep the area clean.

47.   A common cause of a yeast infection in a woman is the kind of condom the man wears during sexual intercourse. Condoms that have a lubricant can cause bacteria that allow yeast infections to form. If this is the case for you, try to use a condom that does not have a spermicidal lubricant.

48.   Wash the vaginal area using a soap that is made for that area. Several different types exist. They will help protect your vagina's natural balance and ensure the area isn't overdried and the flora balance isn't disturbed. Using these rather than regular soaps will keep yeast infections at bay.

49.   Avoid the one-day yeast infection treatments available over the counter. Instead, try a five- or seven-day treatment. The medications in the single

dosage kits are often very strong, and they may lead to further stinging and irritation, on top of that caused by the infection itself. The multi-day treatments are less potent and less likely to be irritating.

50.   There are many foods that can help to fight off yeast infection. One is unsweetened cranberry juice, which can acidify vaginal secretions which in turn will help to kill yeast. Garlic is another popular home remedy, as it has anti-fungal properties. Try two cloves per day in food or salads. Garlic tastes good too!

51.   Taking birth control pills can make many women susceptible to developing a yeast infection. Meanwhile, these pills can prevent unwanted pregnancy; they also aid in the growth of fungi. Many pills contain extensive amounts of estrogen that can upset the balances of nature inside of the vagina. These are the kinds of chances that can lead to yeast infections.

52.   Avoid scented feminine hygiene products. These can cause the pH of your vagina to become imbalanced, which can promote yeast growth. Besides, these products can hide odors that indicate you have an infection.

53.   Yeast infections can cause a discharge that can end up staining your underwear and causing it to develop an odor. You can help combat this problem by wearing a panty-liner in your underwear until your yeast infection has cleared up. This will help to keep your underpants stain free, and also help you to control the odor by changing the pads frequently.

54.   If you like to go to spas and saunas, get your damp clothing off as soon as you are done. Don't wear clothing that is wet because yeast thrives in damp conditions. Dry yourself completely after removing clothes that are wet.

55.   Stay away from douching. You may have the impression that you are cleansing the vagina, but you need the bacterias that you are washing away. When you affect the natural balance of the area, you can be more prone to yeast infections. Cleansing the area with gentle soap and warm water is sufficient.

56.   Avoid wearing underwear while you are at home. Your body needs room to breathe. Yeast infections are more common in the heat. You may feel tempted to wear underwear out of habit. At the very least, however, you should try to begin sleeping

without it. Doing so will make a yeast infection less likely to occur.

57.   Stay away from scented feminine hygiene products. The chemicals used to create those pleasing scents can alter your body's natural pH. This creates an environment that is perfect for a colony of yeast to develop. Bypass the scented pads and tampons and opt for all natural products, free from chemical scents and dyes.

58.   Did you know that the bacteria in plain yogurt can help fight a yeast infection? It is true, but it has to be unsweetened yogurt. Yeast feeds on sugar and yogurt will not be helpful if it contains sugar. You can even use it as a topical treatment by dipping a tampon in yogurt.

59.   One of the big enemies of yeast is garlic. As a home remedy, there is nothing better. Do not use raw garlic, but buy some garlic tablets and insert into the vagina every couple of hours for some soothing relief. Read the label of the garlic tabs and only use the ones that are pure and natural.

60.   Stay away from skinny jeans. Tight fitting pants might look and feel great. Unfortunately, they can also cause yeast infections. Try to avoid them. Instead, wear something thin and airy. You need to

give yourself room to breathe. Keeping your genitals too tightly confined can create the perfect conditions for a yeast infection.

61.   Tight clothing can create an environment prone to yeast infections. Clothes, in particular undergarments which are tight, trap moisture and heat and restrict airflow. Yeast thrives in that sort of damp environment. Try to wear clothing made of natural, breathable fabrics like cotton for example. Ensure they do not fit too tightly.

62.   If you suffer from yeast infections, some changes in your diet may be helpful in keeping them at bay. Try eating yogurt with live cultures that combat yeast. Also, try to eliminate as much sugar as possible from your diet, as sugar has been shown to help yeast to grow.

63.   There are many home remedies available for women to try in order to combat a yeast infection. However, before trying a home remedy, check with your doctor to be certain that what you have is actually a yeast infection. There are other conditions, such as trichomonas and bacterial vaginosis, that can mimic a yeast infection, but require medication to cure.

64.   Even though they are very annoying, yeast infections are also highly treatable. Many drug stores carry over the counter medication to treat yeast infections. If you are not absolutely certain, it is a yeast infection, there are tests that can be done in your doctor's office to determine if that is, in fact, what it is.

65.   Wearing cotton undergarments can help to prevent yeast infections. Cotton is absorbent and non-irritating, unlike some other fabrics. If you suffer from yeast infections often, make sure your underwear is cotton and keep it clean. To absorb the humidity, you can use napkins.

66.   Garlic is a great natural remedy for yeast infection relief and curing. You can apply it two ways. Either you can eat garlic (or foods with garlic), or you can apply it directly to the affected area. If you choose for direct application, make sure to go with pure garlic, preferably all natural and organic, and make sure it is clean. Do not apply more than every three hours.

67.   If you are prone to yeast infections, do not use products like douches, powders or deodorant sprays. These products contain perfumes that can cause yeast infections. If you douche, you could spread the forming yeast infection well into your

uterus and cervix. If the vaginal odor is a problem, talk to your doctor about treatments that do not contain perfumes.

68.   A good tip you can keep in mind if you want to avoid getting a yeast infection is not to wear really tight clothing, especially underwear. The tight clothing will prevent air from getting around your crotch region, and that makes it the perfect breeding ground for a yeast infection.

69.   Eat lots and lots of garlic. Garlic has many benefits, including anti-fungal properties. The anti-fungal properties of garlic can help to prevent and treat yeast infections. However, garlic can thin your blood, so if you are taking any blood thinning medications, consult with your general practitioner before upping your garlic intake.

70.   If you find yourself suffering from chronic yeast infections, you might need to avoid foods that are high in yeast and mold. If your body is already having a difficult time warding off yeast, you don't want to aggravate that condition by consuming more yeast and mold. Foods to avoid would include things like dried fruits, melons, peanuts and most cheeses.

71.   If you wish to keep yeast infections at bay, dry your skin as much as possible after swimming or showering. Moisture is a main cause of common yeast infections. Yeast can grow with water, so make sure that you dry efficiently.

72.   Avoid wearing any clothes that contain irritating or synthetic fibers, as it can be what leads to yeast infections. The infection occurs when clothing is moist or wet, thus providing the perfect thriving environment for the yeast fungus. Consider wearing clothes made from real cotton, as it gives your body room to breathe.

73.   Avoid douching under any circumstances. Although you probably think that douching is a good way to clean your genital area, it is important to realize that the human body has its own self cleaning mechanisms which are delicately balanced. Anything that disrupts the body's natural balance, makes you more prone to an infection. It is enough to clean with water and soap the area.

74.   For a natural way to fight a mild yeast infection, turn to your pantry for a clove of garlic. You can create a suppository with the garlic by nicking it with a knife and inserting it into the vagina overnight. If you are worried about retrieving it, use a needle to pull a piece of string through the clove.

If you experience any irritation, remove the clove promptly.

75.   Be aware that although certain medications may help you, others can increase your chances of getting yeast infections. For instance, when you take an antibiotic when you are sick, you don't only kill bad bacteria you will also kill the good bacteria that will help you fight against yeast infections. If this becomes an issue for you, speak with your doctor.

76.   To help in the prevention of yeast infection, be sure to wear cotton undergarments. Other materials, such as nylon and rayon, hold moisture in, providing an ideal environment for yeast to grow. Cotton stays drier, and keeps moisture away, making the skin less vulnerable to the growth of yeast.

77.   One of the big enemies of yeast is garlic. As a home remedy, there is nothing better. Do not use raw garlic, but buy some garlic tablets and insert into the vagina every couple of hours for some soothing relief. Read the label of the garlic tabs and only use the ones that are pure and natural.

78.   Add some sugar free yogurt as well as garlic to your daily diet. Garlic can help reduce the yeast and prevent infections. If you do not like the taste of

garlic, you can consume garlic pills from your pharmacy. Including sixteen ounces of unsweetened yogurt, with live probiotic cultures, to your diet can significantly minimize occurrences.

79.   An important tip for preventing the occurrence of yeast infections is to avoid lingering in a wet bathing suit for a prolonged period of time. By getting out of wet swimsuits as soon as possible after swimming, you have the power to deprive yeast of the warm, damp environment in which they thrive.

80.   If you are struggling with a yeast infection, try using some plain yogurt. Yogurt contains good bacteria that can fight off the infection. It has to be unsweetened and unflavored since sugar can worsen the infection. You can either apply it via a dipped tampon or you can rub it into the afflicted area.

81.   A major cause of yeast infections is the way you wipe when you have a bowel movement. When you wipe from back to front, you are transferring bacteria from the rectum to the vagina. These bacterias increase your chances of developing a yeast infection. Always wipe from front to back.

82.   It is important to wear loose-fitting clothes to help treat and prevent yeast infections. Yeast

infections are more likely to occur, and irritation during an infection will increase if your clothes are too tight. Consider avoiding such garments as tight jeans, pantyhose and leggings until your yeast infection goes away.

83.   Avoid the one-day yeast infection treatments available over the counter. Instead, try a five- or seven-day treatment. The medications in the single dosage kits are often very strong, and they may lead to further stinging and irritation, on top of that caused by the infection itself. The multi-day treatments are less potent and less likely to be irritating.

84.   Apple cider vinegar can help with yeast infections. Consider adding it to your bath water and sitting in the bath for at least fifteen minutes. The apple cider vinegar can help to restore balance to the vaginal area and bring an end to painful and uncomfortable yeast infection symptoms.

85.   When infected, understand that saliva carries bacteria in excess. If you are infected, it is important to use disposable forks, spoon and paper cups so that you do not spread the condition. Also, disinfect or purchase a new toothbrush to prevent recurring infection. You also need to avoid kissing anyone for a week after your infection has disappeared.

86.	When you go swimming, make sure that you take off your wet suit as soon as possible. Leaving the wet suit on will make you more susceptible to yeast infections. Yeast thrive in moist warm areas, so do your best to make sure they have no way to grow more.

87.	Taking antibiotics for a long period of time can cause you to develop yeast infections. If this happens to you, you should immediately stop taking your antibiotics and contact your doctor. If you have developed yeast infections during the past because of antibiotics, you should let your doctor know about it before he or she prescribes you antibiotics.

88.	If you notice that you are not getting enough sleep, make sure that you are getting at least eight hours per day. This can also be broken down into naps as the day wears on, as sleep will help to get your body back to the functional level to prevent infections all around.

89.	Avoid douching or washing inside of the vagina, as it not only kills off harmful bacteria, but also good ones. Taking douching one step too far can also wash away the protective lining of the vagina, which leaves you more prone to yeast as well as other types of vaginal infections.

90.   Be aware that although certain medications may help you, others can increase your chances of getting yeast infections. For instance, when you take an antibiotic when you are sick, you don't only kill bad bacteria you will also kill the good bacteria that will help you fight against yeast infections. If this becomes an issue for you, speak with your doctor.

91.   Avoid wearing sweaty leotards, leggings, gym clothes or swimsuits any longer than necessary. Because these fabrics are often synthetic, they tend to trap heat and moisture against the skin, which encourages yeast growth. Change into dry clothes as soon as you have the chance; ideally, choose something made from cotton, silk, linen or another breathable fabric.

92.   Get out of your sweaty work clothes as soon as you are able. Dampness can worsen or even cause yeast infections. If you are someone who works out, be sure to change out of your exercise clothes as soon as possible. Take a shower and dry off thoroughly before changing into something else.

93.   A fantastic and natural cure for yeast infections is oil of oregano. You will probably have to go to a

specialty health food store to find it, but it is worth its weight in gold. You need to take this internally and according to the package directions. Find a product that has high levels of carvacrol, which is the active ingredient.

94.   Be aware of the impact of birth control pills. Not only do they help prevent pregnancy, but birth control pills usually contain estrogen as well. Taking estrogen in this way can cause fluctuations in the vagina's natural balance. When this occurs, the environment for yeast growth can be created. If infections are common for you, consult with your physician about options that can help.

95.   If you tend to get yeast infections, your diet should regularly include probiotics. Acidophilus can help balance your body from the inside out, which can help you become more healthy. You can buy probiotic supplements, too.

96.   Be aware that your hormone levels can affect the amount of and intensity of yeast infections. When hormone levels are not stabilized, bad bacteria in the vaginal area is more likely to let in a yeast infection. A number of factors can affect your hormones, such as birth control pills and steroid-based medications, so speak with your doctor about what can be done.

97.   If you suffer from yeast infections, some changes in your diet may be helpful in keeping them at bay. Try eating yogurt with live cultures that combat yeast. Also, try to eliminate as much sugar as possible from your diet, as sugar has been shown to help yeast to grow.

98.   Avoid wearing any nylon pantyhose, especially if you have a career path that requires it. If you must wear pantyhose to work, make sure that you choose one that has a cotton panel to absorb any and all moisture. Always quickly remove your pantyhose after work or opt for thigh high hosiery instead.

99.   After you use the restroom, make sure to wipe yourself from front to back. Wiping back to front can bring bacteria to the vaginal area, and this can cause many infections, including yeast infections. Wiping from front to back helps to keep this region of the body healthy and safe from harmful bacteria.

100.   If you tend to get yeast infection more than once a year, you should consider making changes to your life. Stop taking birth control pills, eliminate foods too rich in sugar and carbs from your diet and improve your hygiene. Schedule an appointment with your doctor and find a solution to get rid of your infections for good.

101.   When treating a yeast infection with creams or suppositories, do not depend on a diaphragm or a condom for birth control. These medications often contain oils that can weaken the latex of barrier forms of birth control. Use an alternate form of protection until you are finished with the course of treatment.

102.   A great tip to help prevent yeast infections from occurring is to keep your showers and/or baths shorter and with warm water instead of hot. Yeast organisms thrive in hotter, moister environments so a long hot shower can greatly increase the chances that you will end up developing a yeast infection.

103.   When you go swimming, make sure that you take off your wet suit as soon as possible. Leaving the wet suit on will make you more susceptible to yeast infections. Yeast thrive in moist warm areas, so do your best to make sure they have no way to grow more.

104.   Don't wear synthetic clothing. Synthetic clothing often traps in moisture leading to the development or worsening of a yeast infection. Instead wear cotton clothing. Cotton clothing allows air to circulate through your clothing to your body, and it

traps in moisture so that your body will remain drier. This will make you less prone to infection.

105.   When you are in the shower, make sure that you wash all of the parts of your body well with soap and water to reduce the amount of bacteria on your skin. Going a day without washing can fester bacteria, which can increase the chances of you getting a serious infection.

106.   If you have a yeast infection, try to reduce the hot and spicy foods that you eat during your meals and snacks. These types of foods can aggravate the infections that you have any make you feel very uncomfortable. Eat moderate foods if you want to feel comfortable with a yeast infection.

107.   Make sure that you practice proper hygiene during a vaginal yeast infection. Always opt to wear cotton panties as synthetic fibers can irritate the infection and make it worse. The infected area should be properly cleaned and kept dry, hence making cotton panties the best option for keeping the area dry.

108.   Only use gentle, non-irritating products on your vagina, avoiding scents. Perfumed sprays and soaps can irritate the area and promote the development of a yeast infection. It is very important to avoid

using scented tampons because they come in direct contact with your vagina. Also avoid the dyes in colored toilet paper.

109.   Avoid wearing sweaty leotards, leggings, gym clothes or swimsuits any longer than necessary. Because these fabrics are often synthetic, they tend to trap heat and moisture against the skin, which encourages yeast growth. Change into dry clothes as soon as you have the chance; ideally, choose something made from cotton, silk, linen or another breathable fabric.

110.   Make sure that you are getting enough sleep each night. Your immune system is what keeps the growth of yeast at bay. By taking the precautions to get enough sleep each night, you are letting your immune system do its job. This means, avoid drinking any caffeine or exercising three hours before bedtime.

111.   A great natural remedy for yeast infections is tea tree oil. Mix several drops of this oil with some sweet almond oil. It can be put right on the affected area. Do not apply tea tree oil straight out of the bottle. If it is not mixed with a carrier oil, it can cause painful burning. This natural remedy is effective in both combating an infection and restoring order to vaginal chemistry.

112.   Yeastarol is a popular yeast infection cure spray that works for both men and women. It is a perfectly natural anti-yeast spray made from all nature derived ingredients. This spray is one of the only all natural yeast infection remedies available on the market today for both men and women.

113.   If you are struggling with a yeast infection, try using some plain yogurt. Yogurt contains good bacteria that can fight off the infection. It has to be unsweetened and unflavored since sugar can worsen the infection. You can either apply it via a dipped tampon or you can rub it into the afflicted area.

114.   Keep you diabetes under good control in order to avoid yeast infections. If you have a blood sugar, infections will be able to thrive in your body. If you have diabetes and suddenly find yourself plagued by recurring yeast infections, this is a good indicator that your blood sugars are out of control.

115.   Eating plenty of plain, unsweetened yogurt is a very good way to prevent and treat yeast infections. The bacteria contained in yogurt will fight off the yeast infection. You can also apply a small amount of yogurt on the infected area and wait a few minutes before washing it off.

116.   When purchasing over-the-counter yeast infection medication, choose a kit with both internal and external medications, along with panty liners. The internal medication will help to cure the infection, and the external cream provides relief from the itching and discomfort until the infection is under control. The panty liners will keep your clothing and underwear clean and mess-free.

117.   Garlic will appease the itching and the burning of a yeast infection. Eating garlic should help prevent yeast infections, but you can also apply a small clove of garlic on the infected area to make the itching disappear. Wash thoroughly after applying the garlic and repeat as often as necessary.

118.   Curing a yeast infection does not have to take a long time. There are several very effective one day treatments available. These can be purchased over the counter at your local pharmacy or supermarket. Give one a try and see if it offers the relief you need from that troublesome infection.

119.   Avoid the one-day yeast infection treatments available over the counter. Instead, try a five- or seven-day treatment. The medications in the single dosage kits are often very strong, and they may lead to further stinging and irritation, on top of that caused by the infection itself. The multi-day

treatments are less potent and less likely to be irritating.

120.   Clean, but do not douche. Don't forget to keep your vaginal area clean while in the shower. Lightly clean it, don't forget the folds. This will help prevent the growth of yeast in moist and warm crevices. Douching may in fact result in infection.

121.   If you have a yeast infection, and have sex with another person, it is important to treat both partners. Yeast infections are transferable between any two individuals (even men). If a partner is dealing with an infection, it best to use a condom to prevent the spread of the infection.

122.   Not only is it important that you wash well to prevent yeast infections, but it is important that you also thoroughly dry the genital area. Yeast tends to form in areas that are moist or damp, especially near the vagina. If you have a hard time getting rid of excess moisture with a towel, do not be afraid to use a blow dryer and a low, cool setting.

123.   If you are taking oral medication for a yeast infection there are some dietary guidelines that can help your body as it fights the infection. First, do not drink alcohol as this will inhibit the medication's effectiveness. The elimination of alcohol will help

ensure that you get the maximum impact from your medication, quickly and on the first round of treatment.

124.   Talk to your doctor about your medications. If you suffer from frequent yeast infections, one of your medications may be to blame. A recent course of antibiotics is a common cause of yeast infections because it kills both the good and bad vaginal bacteria. Birth control or steroids could be another factor.

125.   A great home remedy for relief of the symptoms of a yeast infection is apple cider vinegar. Be careful to never apply straight vinegar to your vagina, it will kill the yeast but will very painful. Putting about a cup and a half in your bathwater for a nice hot soak will bring instant relief.

126.   If you are prone to frequent yeast infections, you should consider taking a supplement that contains additional beneficial bacteria. These bacteria balance your bodies good and bad microorganisms. They are often called prebiotics and probiotics in the stores. Ask the professional at the health food store which one they recommend to balance your bodies microbial system.

127. Keep cool. Yeast tends to thrive in warm environments. Try to keep your vaginal area cool and dry by not taking long hot baths. Also avoid soaking in hot tubs. When the weather is warm, be especially conscious of the clothes that you wear. Don't wear anything too tight that will keep air from cooling your vaginal area.

128. A key tip in prevent yeast infections is to dry yourself thoroughly after each shower. This is due to that fact that yeast will thrive in a moist environment so making sure that you are totally dry after each shower should help you prevent any future yeast infections that may occur.

129. Simple daily routines, such as wearing smooth, cotton underwear can help prevent the occurrence of a yeast infection. Cotton wards off moisture and doesn't irritate the skin. If you tend to get yeast infections often, you should purchase different underwear and make an effort to keep them clean. Protective napkins can also absorb humidity.

130. It is important that you get to the bottom of what is causing your reoccurring yeast infections. Meanwhile, it may not be easy to figure out what the problem is at first. You have to take an objective look at how you're doing things. Diet,

birth control, sexual encounters and clothing may be the cause of yeast infections.

131.   Although it may seem counterintuitive, avoid vaginal wash to prevent yeast infections. Vaginal wash products are often scented and can be irritating. Using these on an ongoing basis can upset the natural balance of the good bacteria in your body. Sometimes chronic vaginal wash use can even completely destroy your healthy natural bacteria.

132.   If you suffer from yeast infections on a regular basis, consider visiting your doctor and getting checked for diabetes. The excess sugar that is often associated with diabetes can cause yeast infections too. A simple urine check can rule out problems, or help you to seek treatment if diabetes is the culprit.

133.   Try to keep your stress levels at bay! Many people who experience an onslaught of stress, often reach for unhealthy junk foods. This also means, more sugar added to an already unhealthy diet. By choosing healthier foods and cutting down stress, you are lowering your chances of developing a yeast infection.

134.   Use garlic aplenty if you are battling off a yeast infection. Garlic supplements are an odor-free way

to keep yeast at bay. These tabs can also be directly inserted into your vagina during infection.

135.   Don't use tampons with scents. They smell great but lead to irritation. This irritation can lead to painful yeast infections that are difficult to get rid of. Only use sanitary products that are unscented.

136.   Consider visiting your doctor. If you are experiencing yeast infections regularly, do not just keep treating it with over the counter medications. Make an appointment with your doctor. It is important that you figure out what is causing your yeast infections and begin taking measures to prevent them from reoccurring.

137.   Men who develop yeast infections are often confused and do not know what to do to cure the problem. Often associated with women, men do not have yeast infections as often as women, but they do have them. Use a tea tree oil powder directly on the penis to clear up a male yeast infection.

138.   If you have diabetes, keep your sugar under control. Uncontrolled blood sugar can increase your risk of all kinds of infections, including yeast infections. If you experience frequent yeast infections, talk about your options with your

doctor. You may need a prophylactic course of anti-fungal medications until your diabetes is better-controlled.

139.   When you go swimming, take off your wet swimsuit as soon as you are finished. Do not spend any more time in damp clothing than you have to, because it creates an ideal environment for yeast growth. To avoid excess moisture in the vaginal area, remove wet clothing immediately and thoroughly dry the area before putting on fresh clothes.

140.   Did you know that the bacteria in plain yogurt can help fight a yeast infection? It is true, but it has to be unsweetened yogurt. Yeast feeds on sugar and yogurt will not be helpful if it contains sugar. You can even use it as a topical treatment by dipping a tampon in yogurt.

141.   A great home remedy for relief of the symptoms of a yeast infection is apple cider vinegar. Be careful to never apply straight vinegar to your vagina, it will kill the yeast but will very painful. Putting about a cup and a half in your bathwater for a nice hot soak will bring instant relief.

142.   Take a look at your diet if you keep getting yeast infections. Too much sugar intake can create the

optimal breeding ground for yeast infections. If diet turns out to be the culprit, consider substituting fruit for other sugary snacks.

143.   If you have a yeast infection, you need to stop taking your birth control pills until it passes. The birth control pills will weaken your immune system and actually prevent your body from fighting it off. So try using alternative forms of contraception like condoms when you are having a yeast infection.

144.   Douching is a common cause of yeast infections. Though they are sold as a cleansing product, douches can actually encourage yeast infections. The natural bacterial that your body produces will be upset when you douche. When the good bacteria is removed from your vagina, it leaves room for yeast infections to occur.

145.   To help prevent yeast infections avoid scratches. Even tiny lacerations can lead to a yeast infection. Scratches can be caused by sex, or even tampons. Be careful when it comes to both activities. If frequent yeast infections plague you, avoid rough or vigorous sexual activity.

146.   A yeast infection in your mouth can be frightening. It often happens in infants, but can happen in adults as well. The best ways to fight an

oral yeast infection is to rinse your mouth with warm salt water and avoid eating sugar. The salt water will flush out some yeast and not eating sugar will starve the yeast.

147.   Yeast infection can really get out of control before you know it. While there are over the counter methods of ridding yourself of a yeast infection, it's imperative that you also see a doctor. Make sure you are completely aware of your situation and getting rid of the yeast infection as soon as possible.

148.   Taking birth control pills can make many women susceptible to developing a yeast infection. Meanwhile, these pills can prevent unwanted pregnancy; they also aid in the growth of fungi. Many pills contain extensive amounts of estrogen that can upset the balances of nature inside of the vagina. These are the kinds of chances that can lead to yeast infections.

149.   Your underwear should be made of quality cotton. If the underwear are not made of cotton, make sure that there is at least a panel in the crotch that is cotton. Keep your underwear clean and dry. Yeast will grow in damp environments, so if you sweat or leak a bit, change your underwear as soon as possible.

150.   There are many over-the-counter treatments that work well with yeast infections. These include Ticonazole, Miconazole, Butoconazole and Clotrimazole. Use them by gently massaging it into the affected area for the amount of days recommended in the directions. However, it is important to avoid these products if you are currently pregnant.

151.   Try to reduce your stress levels. Too much stress can weaken your immune system and leave you more susceptible to yeast infections. Try to avoid stress as a preventative measure. If you are currently suffering from a yeast infection, remaining too stressed out might exacerbate your infection. Practice some calming activities.

152.   Avoid wearing tight clothes so that your crotch area can get proper air circulation. This is because yeast thrives in hot and moist climates that can occur when you wear this type of clothing.

153.   The garments you wear can create an environment that is friendly to bacteria, and can invite a yeast infection. Make sure to wear loose fitting under and outer garments, especially in warm weather. Underwear with a cotton crotch is

recommended in all seasons, but is more important when the weather is warm.

154.   Diabetics may find that they are much more prone to contracting yeast infections. Men and women alike, will find that they have to work extra hard to control their blood sugar levels. Make sure to try to keep your blood sugar levels as close to normal as possible in order to prevent any infections.

155.   Don't self-diagnose. If you are unsure of whether you have a yeast infection, it is best to visit your doctor. Other sexually transmitted diseases can have similar symptoms, but if not treated properly, can cause serious complications in the long run. It is best to verify that it is a yeast infection, especially if you're pregnant or this is your first experience with an infection.

156.   Know what the symptoms of a yeast infection are. Before you ever have a yeast infection, it is a smart idea to know what symptoms are. Why? Because when you know the symptoms, you can better deal with the infection more quickly so that it does not become a bigger problem.

157.   The best way to prevent yeast infections is to dress properly. Cotton and silk are natural fibers

that absorb moisture and will help keep the area dry. Nylon and other man made fabrics will not absorb moisture as well, and you will increase the likelihood of getting a yeast infection.

158.   Stepping up your personal hygiene habits can help to prevent recurring yeast infections. After using the bathroom, you should avoid wiping from back to font. Instead, you should do the reverse. This prevents the spread of bacteria and yeast that might otherwise be transferred from the anal area to the vagina. Wiping properly and thoroughly can save you a great deal of discomfort.

159.   There are certain foods you can avoid eating to prevent yeast infections. Candida is a trigger of yeast infections and it thrives on foods that are high in sugar, yeast, caffeine, sulphates and moldy foods, like dairy products. Avoiding these foods will increase your chances of avoiding yeast infections altogether.

160.   Fighting yeast infections is made easier with a little yogurt. Yogurt applied directly to the vaginal area can soothe discomfort and help balance to return to a woman's body. Yogurt contains Lactobacillus Acidophilus, and this is found in a healthy vagina. Make sure the yogurt is plain, and use a pad to help prevent messes.

161.   One of the big enemies of yeast is garlic. As a home remedy, there is nothing better. Do not use raw garlic, but buy some garlic tablets and insert into the vagina every couple of hours for some soothing relief. Read the label of the garlic tabs and only use the ones that are pure and natural.

162.   Get out of your sweaty work clothes as soon as you are able. Dampness can worsen or even cause yeast infections. If you are someone who works out, be sure to change out of your exercise clothes as soon as possible. Take a shower and dry off thoroughly before changing into something else.

163.   If you suspect that you have a yeast infection, and you have never had one before, see your doctor. He or she can give you an accurate diagnosis. This is important, because there are other serious infections that can mimic the symptoms of a yeast infection. Treating the wrong infection will prolong your misery and could lead to long-term problems for your reproductive system.

164.   Drink cranberry juice to treat your yeast infection. This juice is great for urinary tract issues, but it can effectively treat yeast infections too. It will help flush out the bacteria and fungi that is causing the infection. Drinking a couple of cups a

day for a couple of weeks can help get rid of the discomfort and infection.

165.   Antibiotics can cause yeast infections. While antibiotics are very beneficial and even lifesaving, they can kill the beneficial bacteria in the vaginal area. The result is sometimes a troublesome yeast infection. Consider speaking with your doctor to lower the amount of time you are on the antibiotic if possible and reduce your risk of a yeast infection.

166.   Always watch where you're wiping. Any time you use the bathroom, but especially after a bowel movement, it is important to remember to wipe from front to back instead of back to front. If you wipe from back to front, you risk transferring yeast and fecal bacteria to your vagina, which can cause infections.

167.   It has been debated for many years, but it can be said that many women who have sexual intercourse will suffer from a yeast infection. While yeast infections are not categorized under sexually transmitted infections, it is still shown that 12% of men get yeast infections from women who already have a yeast infection.

168.   If you are suffering from yeast infections, consider making changes to your diet. Diets high in

sugar and processed foods offer the perfect environment inside the body for yeast. Sometimes finding the solution is as easy as reducing processed foods and sugars, and consuming a whole food diet instead.

169.   If you want to prevent yeast infections, you should try to incorporate yogurt into your diet. Live culture yogurt is the best for preventing yeast infections. The yogurt needs to be sugar free in order for it to be effective. If you do get a yeast infection, you can use sugar free yogurt as a topical cream as well.

170.   People get yeast infections when the pH balance of their vaginas is thrown off. You can mess up this balance by consuming things like beer and certain fruits. One way to keep your pH in check is to eat yogurt on a regular basis. This helps keep things under control.

171.   Many people may not know this, but having an excessive intake of sugar in their diets can in fact, result in yeast infections. Take preventative care and limit the amount of sugar you have in your diet. Make sure that you eat a healthy and balanced meal that evens out all the bad things.

172.   Taking acidophilus tablets regularly can prevent yeast infections. Acidophilus is a naturally occurring enzyme that keeps your body maintain the proper pH-balance. This helps to prevent yeast infections because they are often brought on by an imbalance of bacteria in the body.

173.   Cinnamon is a wonderful herb that can help reduce the effects of infection if you happen to catch a yeast infection. You can sprinkle a little amount of cinnamon on many different things, whether you are using it on a meal or dessert to help reduce the chances of infection in your body.

174.   After you go swimming, you need to change into dry clothes as soon as possible. Wearing a wet bikini bottom is a big cause of yeast infections. Moisture is a breeding ground for yeast. If you cannot change or do not have dry clothes, use a blow dryer on a cool setting to dry the area and your suit.

175.   For a natural way to fight a mild yeast infection, turn to your pantry for a clove of garlic. You can create a suppository with the garlic by nicking it with a knife and inserting it into the vagina overnight. If you are worried about retrieving it, use a needle to pull a piece of string through the clove.

If you experience any irritation, remove the clove promptly.

176.   One tip that you should follow after you go to the bathroom is to always wipe from the front side to the back side to prevent the spread of bacteria. Follow this technique to prevent any spread of bacteria, which is one of the main causes of yeast infections forming in your body.

177.   Not only is it important that you wash well to prevent yeast infections, but it is important that you also thoroughly dry the genital area. Yeast tends to form in areas that are moist or damp, especially near the vagina. If you have a hard time getting rid of excess moisture with a towel, do not be afraid to use a blow dryer and a low, cool setting.

178.   Avoid synthetic fibers and tight clothing. Tight clothing, especially underwear, traps moisture and raises your body temperature, as well as constricting airflow. Yeast thrives in the warm, moist environment that develops when air is unable to circulate. On your next shopping trip, opt for clothing and undergarments made of natural fibers, such as cotton, and avoid tight clothing.

179.   Take a look at your diet if yeast infections are a recurring issue. Eating a lot of high-sugar foods

makes it much easier for yeast to grow in your system. If your poor dietary habits are causing the yeast infections, try to switch from sugary foods to nuts, veggies, and fruits.

180.   In order to avoid and treat yeast infections, drink fresh cranberry juice. Fresh cranberries have a natural ingredient that is a preventative and cure for yeast infections. Try to drink a little bit of cranberry juice every day to ward off yeast infections. If you already have a yeast infection, increase your daily cranberry intake to help ease the symptoms.

181.   Do not wear tight pants, particular really skinny jeans. These jeans do not give your crotch air, which can be detrimental to your vaginal health. Yeast infections develop in warm, moist environments with little circulation. To reduce your risk, wear loose-fitting clothing.

182.   Eat yogurt daily in order to prevent yeast infections. The healthy bacteria contained in yogurt helps your body to ward off a build-up of yeast. Eating yogurt on a regular basis enables your system to kill the fungus that causes yeast infections. If you already have a yeast infection, you can eat yogurt or even apply plain yogurt topically to help soothe the symptoms.

183.   Take steps to boost your immune system if you are prone to chronic yeast infections. If your body's defenses are strong, you will be better able to ward off yeast infections. Therefore, try to improve your overall health. Exercise more, quit smoking, take a multivitamin and avoid sweets to help improve your body's immune system and avoid yeast infections.

184.   Avoid wearing synthetic fibers. Synthetic materials trap moisture and prevent air circulation. Yeast loves that type of environment. So, when you avoid this kind of clothing, you are reducing the chances of yeast infections.

185.   Garlic is a great natural remedy for yeast infection relief and curing. You can apply it two ways. Either you can eat garlic (or foods with garlic), or you can apply it directly to the affected area. If you choose for direct application, make sure to go with pure garlic, preferably all natural and organic, and make sure it is clean. Do not apply more than every three hours.

186.   Steer clear of any sex while you are experiencing a yeast infection. Any sort of sexual relations can lead to the spread of the infection between partners. If this is not a choice, then it is essential that a condom is used. WHile not foolproof, a condom can potentially help the spread of the infection.

187.   Wear clothing constructed of natural materials. Cotton is a great option, because it is natural and absorbs moisture. Synthetic fabrics can cause yeast infections.

188.   One of the most common symptoms of yeast infections is itching and burning. These symptoms take a while to ease up, even after starting on medication. Use cold washcloths and ice packs to relieve the itchiness. Avoid scratching.

189.   If you have a yeast infection, you should remember that garlic can fight effectively against it. Some individuals espose direct application of garlic cloves and tabs directly to their vaginas. Other people prefer to eat the garlic instead. In either case, garlic fans espouse how effective it is at minimizing the itchiness and discomfort of having a yeast infection.

190.   Apple cider vinegar is a great ingredient that you can use to help fight the symptoms when you already have a yeast infection. If you are going to consume this product, make sure that you dilute it heavily with water as you should only be using one teaspoon to drink with.

191.   Go on a special diet to stop recurring yeast infections. Many find that eliminating sugar from their diet and decreasing the grains they consume to be beneficial in curbing a yeast infection. Give these diet considerations a try and they may help you to never have a yeast infection again.

192.   Ibuprofen or aspirin can reduce the pain associated with a yeast infection. Yeast infections are quite painful, so you want to do what you can to mitigate this pain and stay productive.

193.   Get out of your bathing suit as soon as you can, if you want to avoid yeast infections. Excessive moisture can cause a yeast infection to brew, so make sure you change into something dry as soon as you can. When on trips, make sure to bring two bathing suits so that you never have to wear a wet one for too long.

194.   Make sure you dry yourself very thoroughly after bathing and showering to prevent yeast infections. Yeast thrive in moist environments, including folds of skin found almost anywhere on the body. Gently pat the skin dry with an absorbent towel, and then apply body powder to these areas to absorb even more moisture.

195.   Be aware that although certain medications may help you, others can increase your chances of getting yeast infections. For instance, when you take an antibiotic when you are sick, you don't only kill bad bacteria you will also kill the good bacteria that will help you fight against yeast infections. If this becomes an issue for you, speak with your doctor.

196.   As a woman, you may think that douching your vaginal area will help keep you clean; this is actually not true. When you douche, you are stripping the natural protective lining of the vagina, allowing yeast infections to form. Douching also eliminates your body's good bacteria, which leaves you more susceptible to yeast infections.

197.   Keep your vaginal area dry and clean. Yeast infections are more likely to occur if you do not. Be sure to wash regularly. Wear absorbent panties, like cotton. This will help to keep your vaginal area dry throughout the day, thus decreasing the likelihood of you developing a yeast infection.

198.   A common cause of a yeast infection in a woman is the kind of condom the man wears during sexual intercourse. Condoms that have a lubricant can cause bacteria that allow yeast infections to form. If this is the case for you, try to

use a condom that does not have a spermicidal lubricant.

199.   When purchasing over-the-counter yeast infection medication, choose a kit with both internal and external medications, along with panty liners. The internal medication will help to cure the infection, and the external cream provides relief from the itching and discomfort until the infection is under control. The panty liners will keep your clothing and underwear clean and mess-free.

200.   Keep cool. Yeast tends to thrive in warm environments. Try to keep your vaginal area cool and dry by not taking long hot baths. Also avoid soaking in hot tubs. When the weather is warm, be especially conscious of the clothes that you wear. Don't wear anything too tight that will keep air from cooling your vaginal area.

201.   Keep dry. Yeast thrives in a warm, moist environment. After you finish your shower or bath, make sure you dry your crotch area thoroughly. Some women even find a blow dryer on the lowest setting to be useful for this purpose. Never put on any clothing until the area is completely dry.

202.   If you are suffering from yeast infections, consider making changes to your diet. Diets high in

sugar and processed foods offer the perfect environment inside the body for yeast. Sometimes finding the solution is as easy as reducing processed foods and sugars, and consuming a whole food diet instead.

203.   Keep the chemicals you use for personal cleansing to a minimum or less, if you want to avoid yeast infections. Such chemicals will strip your body of its natural PH balance, and ability to control yeast. Check with your doctor to learn what the most effective products are that won't leave you vulnerable.

204.   Choose clothes that contain cotton and other natural materials. Unlike most man-made fibers, natural materials allow the skin to breathe and prevent the buildup of heat and moisture. Moist, humid conditions encourage yeast infections, so it is important to wear breathable clothing.

205.   There are many foods that can contribute to a yeast infection by inhibiting the immune system and allowing yeast to grow. If you suffer from frequent yeast infections, try to avoid foods such as sugar, cheese, alcohol, mushrooms and milk. On the other hand, foods like yogurt with live cultures can inhibit the overgrowth of yeast.

206.   A good tip to consider if you'd like to avoid getting a yeast infection is to make sure you dry yourself very thoroughly after swimming or taking a bath. Yeast infections love dampness and moisture, so incomplete drying can cause a risk.

207.   Overcoming a yeast infection can sometimes be as easy as adjusting your diet. It has been shown that sugar can promote the development of yeast infections. On the other hand, yogurt has beneficial cultures which can help eliminate infections for good.

208.   One of the ways that you can prevent yeast infections altogether is to limit the alcohol intake that you consume during the day and night. Alcohol can hurt your immune system, which is a very important component in fighting the fungus that can lead to moderate and severe yeast infections.

209.   The kind of underwear you wear plays a major role on whether or not you develop yeast infections. On the one hand, cotton and silky underwear absorb moisture, keeping your vaginal area dry and preventing infections from forming. On the other hand, synthetic fibers, like nylon, pull moisture close to your skin, increasing your chances of a yeast infection.

210.   Treat a mild yeast infection with plain, unsweetened yogurt. You can freeze yogurt in tampon applicators or the fingers of rubber gloves to make easy-to-insert and soothing suppositories. You can also use a syringe to apply the yogurt. Wear a maxi pad with this treatment to keep the mess to a minimum.

211.   Garlic is a great natural remedy, and it has proven effective in fighting yeast infections. Create a garlic tampon by tying string to a couple of cloves and inserting it into the vagina. Leave it in for a couple of hours, and relief will typically come. The antifungal properties of the garlic have a healing effect and can effectively combat troublesome yeast.

212.   Since yeast thrives in moist environments, it is imperative to stay as dry as possible at all times. If you have been swimming, change into dry clothing as quickly as possible. Furthermore, exercise can cause sweat and moisture to build up, so it is important to shower and change into clean underwear and clothing after a workout.

213.   Even though they are very annoying, yeast infections are also highly treatable. Many drug stores carry over the counter medication to treat yeast infections. If you are not absolutely certain, it is a yeast infection, there are tests that can be done

in your doctor's office to determine if that is, in fact, what it is.

214.   Yeast infection can really get out of control before you know it. While there are over the counter methods of ridding yourself of a yeast infection, it's imperative that you also see a doctor. Make sure you are completely aware of your situation and getting rid of the yeast infection as soon as possible.

215.   Do not just assume you have a yeast infection; go to your doctor and have him or her diagnose it. Other infections, such as bacterial vaginosis, have similar symptoms as yeast infections do. It is important that you find out which you have, as the treatment for yeast infections differ from other conditions.

216.   While many people may believe that douching is a good way to prevent the onset of yeast infections this is actually not the case. Douching destroys both harmful as well as helpful bacteria that can help prevent yeast infections from occurring. Do yourself a favor and stay away from douching.

217.   It has been debated for many years, but it can be said that many women who have sexual intercourse will suffer from a yeast infection. While yeast

infections are not categorized under sexually transmitted infections, it is still shown that 12% of men get yeast infections from women who already have a yeast infection.

218.   If you are suffering from yeast infections, consider making changes to your diet. Diets high in sugar and processed foods offer the perfect environment inside the body for yeast. Sometimes finding the solution is as easy as reducing processed foods and sugars, and consuming a whole food diet instead.

219.   To cut down on your chances or impact from a yeast infection, stay thoroughly hydrated. The often you urinate, the more likely you are to flush excess sugars out of your system. This drastically cuts down on both your chances of a yeast infection and the lifespan of any current ones.

220.   If you are breastfeeding and suffering from thrush, a type of yeast infection, make sure to treat both yourself and your baby. If you do not treat both your breasts and your baby's mouth, the yeast will continue to multiply, and you will not find the cure you are looking for.

221.   There are many foods that can contribute to a yeast infection by inhibiting the immune system and

allowing yeast to grow. If you suffer from frequent yeast infections, try to avoid foods such as sugar, cheese, alcohol, mushrooms and milk. On the other hand, foods like yogurt with live cultures can inhibit the overgrowth of yeast.

222.   Try to keep your stress under control. It has not been proven in scientific studies, but many people have observed that stress is linked to yeast infections. If you are often stressed out or have a highly stressful job, try to manage your stress the best you can by using meditation, yoga, or deep breathing.

223.   The burn and itch of a yeast infection is infuriating. These symptoms can linger a lot longer than you want them to. Cold water on a wash cloth, or a sitz bath can help you feel better. It is essential that you do not scratch.

224.   A great tip to consider if you don't want to end up getting a yeast infection is to not linger in really hot environments such as a hot bath. Yeast thrives in hot and wet environments and you're more likely to get a yeast infection if you stay in one for too long.

225.   Eat more yogurt. Eating yogurt will not cure a yeast infection. However, some women have found

that eating a daily yogurt along with their antibiotics can help immensely. Give it a try. With any luck, it could get rid of your yeast infection faster and keep the infection from returning.

226.   Make sure that if you suffer from a yeast infection, you seek natural remedies. Many of the drugs available on the market today contain nasty side effects. Natural remedies can range from yogurt and apple cider to vinegar garlic. There are plenty of other natural solutions available for a yeast infection.

227.   Make sure that you practice proper hygiene during a vaginal yeast infection. Always opt to wear cotton panties as synthetic fibers can irritate the infection and make it worse. The infected area should be properly cleaned and kept dry, hence making cotton panties the best option for keeping the area dry.

228.   The kind of underwear you wear plays a major role on whether or not you develop yeast infections. On the one hand, cotton and silky underwear absorb moisture, keeping your vaginal area dry and preventing infections from forming. On the other hand, synthetic fibers, like nylon, pull moisture close to your skin, increasing your chances of a yeast infection.

229.   Avoid perfumed soaps and bubble baths. The perfumes used on these products can promote yeast infections. Refrain from using tampons that have scents on them as well.

230.   Eat a lot of yogurt if you want to stop yeast infections. Yogurt contains bacteria that work to fight against yeast infections. Bear in mind, however, that most experts believe that eating yogurt does not cure yeast infections that may already exist.

231.   If you have to take antibiotics, be even more alert and proactive towards yeast infections. Antibiotics can kill off all the bacteria in your body, and that includes the good stuff. Try taking extra probiotics or talk to your doctor and ask what he recommends.

232.   There are many foods that can help to fight off yeast infection. One is unsweetened cranberry juice, which can acidify vaginal secretions which in turn will help to kill yeast. Garlic is another popular home remedy, as it has anti-fungal properties. Try two cloves per day in food or salads. Garlic tastes good too!

233.   Do not just assume you have a yeast infection; go to your doctor and have him or her diagnose it. Other infections, such as bacterial vaginosis, have similar symptoms as yeast infections do. It is important that you find out which you have, as the treatment for yeast infections differ from other conditions.

234.   There are many over-the-counter treatments that work well with yeast infections. These include Ticonazole, Miconazole, Butoconazole and Clotrimazole. Use them by gently massaging it into the affected area for the amount of days recommended in the directions. However, it is important to avoid these products if you are currently pregnant.

235.   To cut down on your chances or impact from a yeast infection, stay thoroughly hydrated. The often you urinate, the more likely you are to flush excess sugars out of your system. This drastically cuts down on both your chances of a yeast infection and the lifespan of any current ones.

236.   If you have an infected throat or mouth, your saliva contains yeast bacteria Avoid putting items in your mouth, along with using paper cups and plastic silverware. Make sure to properly clean your toothbrush after each use, and cough into your

elbow, if you must. You should also avoid kissing anyone for 7 days following the infection disappearing.

237.   When you go swimming, make sure that you take off your wet suit as soon as possible. Leaving the wet suit on will make you more susceptible to yeast infections. Yeast thrive in moist warm areas, so do your best to make sure they have no way to grow more.

238.   Those that suffer from diabetes should take extra care to keep their blood sugar levels under control if they wish to prevent a yeast infection from occurring. If your blood sugar is too high, or too low you have a much greater risk of developing a yeast infection than someone with normal blood sugar.

239.   Some studies have shown that a diet consisting of yogurt that contains active cultures can actually combat any overgrowth of yeast. This is good advice to anyone currently has a yeast infection, or simple just wishes to prevent any from occurring. Just make sure that the yogurt you eat has active cultures.

240.   If you find yourself suffering from chronic yeast infections, you might need to avoid foods that are

high in yeast and mold. If your body is already having a difficult time warding off yeast, you don't want to aggravate that condition by consuming more yeast and mold. Foods to avoid would include things like dried fruits, melons, peanuts and most cheeses.

241.   While yeast infections are not considered STIs, be aware that they can be passed between partners in rare cases. If you are comfortable enough to have sex, use a barrier method to prevent passing the infection to a partner. If you are using a cream to treat the infection, use an additional back-up form of protection, because the cream may weaken a condom or diaphragm.

242.   The beneficial bacteria that is found in plain yogurt can be a natural yeast fighter. Yogurt can be applied topically, but some find it a bit messy and prefer to ingest it instead. It is essential that you purchase plain, unsweetened yogurt, because the sugars in sweetened yogurt can actually feed the yeast and cause it to flourish.

243.   If you get frequent yeast infections, you may need to change your bath products. Stay away from any hygiene products that feature dyes or fragrances. These types of items can interfere with the pH balance and internal environment of the

vagina, and can help promote the growth of yeast. You should instead use hypoallergenic and mild products.

244.   Don't use a douche. Your body naturally balances itself. When you disrupt the natural environment, it makes infections more likely. Normal washing with soap and warm water is all that is required.

245.   If you suffer from recurrent yeast infections, try not to wear panty liners, which can irritate your skin and create yeast infections. Try to stick with cotton fiber underwear, as this can provide the most comfortable feeling possible and help to limit the amount of moisture that you have in your area.

246.   In order to prevent yeast infections, especially in women, limit the amount of time you spend in the heat. This means to limit time you spend bathing in hot water. Yeast organisms love hot and moist areas; therefore they thrive. Furthermore, remember to avoid wearing any tight clothing that can stop proper air circulation in the crotch area.

247.   Try tweaking your diet as a way to prevent yeast infections. It is possible that consuming more active cultures by adding probiotic yogurts to your diet may inhibit excessive yeast growth. Another option

to try is reducing your sugar consumption, which is also thought to prevent yeast from growing.

248.   If a yeast infection hits you every time you get a period, start being proactive. Consume a couple of acidophilus tablets prior to the period starting, and a couple when it's over. Your symptoms will decrease in severity or disappear altogether. By taking such steps to help yourself, you may not have to worry about yeast infections any more.

249.   Keep you diabetes under good control in order to avoid yeast infections. If you have a blood sugar, infections will be able to thrive in your body. If you have diabetes and suddenly find yourself plagued by recurring yeast infections, this is a good indicator that your blood sugars are out of control.

250.   Avoid wearing any nylon pantyhose, especially if you have a career path that requires it. If you must wear pantyhose to work, make sure that you choose one that has a cotton panel to absorb any and all moisture. Always quickly remove your pantyhose after work or opt for thigh high hosiery instead.

251.   Try eating more garlic. Adding a little more garlic to your diet can do wonders if you suffer from yeast infections. Studies have found that garlic has the ability to kill off yeast. This can be used to

get rid of yeast infections and may prevent them from reoccurring in the future.

252.   For a natural home remedy to a yeast infection, consider apple-cider vinegar. Drinking apple-cider vinegar and apply it externally both provide relief. But, because it has the ability to cause burning, topical use may be risky. Rather, consider adding a few cups of apple cider vinegar to warm bathwater.

253.   Know the differences between yeast infections and bacterial infections. A yeast infection causes itching, burning, redness and discharge that looks like cottage cheese. Bacterial infections cause foul smells, itching, irritation and discharge that may appear yellowish or greenish in color. If you aren't sure which type you have, seek medical attention before attempting treatment.

254.   People get yeast infections when the pH balance of their vaginas is thrown off. You can mess up this balance by consuming things like beer and certain fruits. One way to keep your pH in check is to eat yogurt on a regular basis. This helps keep things under control.

255.   If you have a mild yeast infection right before your period is supposed to start, you may be able to wait it out. The pH of the vagina becomes

unsuitable for yeast growth when your period begins, and it will probably clear up on its own. This can be very uncomfortable in the meantime, however.

256.   Apple cider vinegar is great to help cure and relieve the symptoms of a yeast infection. While you can put it directly on the vagina, it will burn like crazy. Instead, add a cup or so to a hot bath. It will help kill the yeast and relieve the itching.

257.   If you want to avoid yeast infections, make sure you are getting enough sleep. When you are properly rested, your immune system can probably fight off yeast infections on its own. Avoid caffeine and exercise in the three hours prior to going to bed, and get the same seven to nine hours every night.

258.   If you experience four or more yeast infections in a year outside of antibiotic use, see your doctor. Self-treatment may not be appropriate for frequent or recurring yeast infections. There could be an underlying disorder that is causing the yeast growth, and it's best to find the root cause, if possible.

259.   Homemade remedies and natural cures are very efficient against yeast infections. There are several natural products which can help to both prevent

and treat yeast infections, including live culture yogurt, garlic and more. You also won't have to deal with any side effects.

260.   To avoid yeast infections, avoid using anything scented regarding your vagina. Any scented material, or even a scent itself, can upset the pH balance of this part of your body. That leaves it far more susceptible to a yeast infection. If you have one already, it makes it harder to fight off.

261.   The best way to avoid yeast infections is to clean yourself thoroughly. If you keep your vagina clean, you will help prevent yeast infections. Clean the inside folds because that is where yeast infections are more likely to grow. Usually with proper hygiene, you can prevent yeast infections from occurring.

262.   The best way to prevent yeast infections is to dress properly. Cotton and silk are natural fibers that absorb moisture and will help keep the area dry. Nylon and other man made fabrics will not absorb moisture as well, and you will increase the likelihood of getting a yeast infection.

263.   Check the deodorant that you are using if you continually get yeast infections as the year progresses. Deodorants can have chemicals in them

that may impact the formation of fungus on and in your body. Switch deodorants or go to your doctor for a prescription grade deodorant if you feel this may be the culprit.

264.   If you are prone to yeast infections, always wear underwear made from 100 percent cotton fabric, or at least make sure the crotch is cotton. Polyester and other synthetic fabrics can trap moisture, which allows yeast to thrive. Because cotton is breathable, it leaves you feeling drier and does not contribute to a yeast-friendly environment.

265.   Some medications can actually increase your risk for getting yeast infections. In a recent study, it was shown the antibiotics used for bladder infections kill not only harmful bacteria, but also helpful ones that help control yeast production. Taking oral steroids and/or birth control pills can also increase your chances of developing a yeast infection.

266.   As a woman, you may think that douching your vaginal area will help keep you clean; this is actually not true. When you douche, you are stripping the natural protective lining of the vagina, allowing yeast infections to form. Douching also eliminates your body's good bacteria, which leaves you more susceptible to yeast infections.

267.   To help in the prevention of yeast infection, be sure to wear cotton undergarments. Other materials, such as nylon and rayon, hold moisture in, providing an ideal environment for yeast to grow. Cotton stays drier, and keeps moisture away, making the skin less vulnerable to the growth of yeast.

268.   You should shun wearing tight clothes and garments made from synthetic fabrics. Tight clothing restricts airflow and keeps moisture and heat from escaping. Yeast grows in damp, warm environments, and low airflow sets the stage for that kind of environment. Wear clothes made from cotton or other fabric that provides good ventilation, and be sure that the clothes are not overly tight.

269.   If you have recurring yeast infections, review what you usually eat. Sugar, in particular, encourages the growth of yeast. If you discover that poor eating habits may be contributing to your yeast infections, try switching out sugary snacks with fruits, vegetables and nuts instead.

270.   A major cause of yeast infections is the way you wipe when you have a bowel movement. When you wipe from back to front, you are transferring bacteria from the rectum to the vagina. These

bacterias increase your chances of developing a yeast infection. Always wipe from front to back.

271.   Eat more garlic or take garlic supplements to help avoid yeast infections. Garlic contains a natural ingredient that kills yeast. Consuming more garlic boost your body's ability to control the yeast in your system and ward off yeast infections. If you already have a yeast infection, you can also use garlic to soothe the symptoms.

272.   If you are trying to keep yeast infections away, consider adding garlic and fresh cranberries to your diet. These foods contain natural anti-fungul agents. When ingested, they can help to keep your entire body healthy. Adding a serving of each to your daily diet just might be enough to keep the yeast infections away.

273.   Take antibiotics with caution if you are prone to yeast infections. Antibiotics are the most common medicine-related cause of yeast infections so make sure you really need the medicine, or risk the consequences. Have a fast acting remedy on hand for yeast infections when ever you have to take antibiotics.

274.   You can prevent yeast infections by improving your hygiene. Wash your vagina with a special soap:

choose a product with a neutral PH if possible and douche once a week. Use mouthwash and floss to get rid of the bacteria present in your mouth. Use a clean towel to dry after showering.

275.   Antibiotics can cause yeast infections. While antibiotics are very beneficial and even lifesaving, they can kill the beneficial bacteria in the vaginal area. The result is sometimes a troublesome yeast infection. Consider speaking with your doctor to lower the amount of time you are on the antibiotic if possible and reduce your risk of a yeast infection.

276.   To relieve the burning and itching of a yeast infection, apply the juice from an aloe vera plant. You can also apply the juice to a cotton pad, place it in the fridge, and apply the cool liquid for soothing relief. Note that the aloe does not fight the yeast--it merely soothes the external symptoms.

277.   Pure organic vinegar can be very effective in treating the symptoms of a common yeast infection. Vinegar is very strong so applying it directly to the affected area is not recommended. Instead, add a cup of vinegar to your bath water and relax in the bath for temporary relief of symptoms.

278.   People get yeast infections when the pH balance of their vaginas is thrown off. You can mess up this

balance by consuming things like beer and certain fruits. One way to keep your pH in check is to eat yogurt on a regular basis. This helps keep things under control.

279.   Get out of your bathing suit as soon as you can, if you want to avoid yeast infections. Excessive moisture can cause a yeast infection to brew, so make sure you change into something dry as soon as you can. When on trips, make sure to bring two bathing suits so that you never have to wear a wet one for too long.

280.   Avoid douching or washing inside of the vagina, as it not only kills off harmful bacteria, but also good ones. Taking douching one step too far can also wash away the protective lining of the vagina, which leaves you more prone to yeast as well as other types of vaginal infections.

281.   Limit your intake of sugar during an infection. Yeast thrives on the presence of sugar, and sugar is found in much of your diet if you are not vigilant. Cheeses and other dairy, breads and alcohol are some of the primary sources of sugars that yeast will consume in an effort to flourish.

282.   Start eating yogurt. That's right, the next time you feel the itching and burning that comes with

yeast infections, grab yourself a cup of yogurt. Acidophilus, a healthy bacteria, is contained in yogurt. This healthy bacteria can help fight off a yeast infection and will make it go away quicker.

283.   Stay away from skinny jeans. Tight fitting pants might look and feel great. Unfortunately, they can also cause yeast infections. Try to avoid them. Instead, wear something thin and airy. You need to give yourself room to breathe. Keeping your genitals too tightly confined can create the perfect conditions for a yeast infection.

284.   If you tend to get yeast infections, monitor what you eat. Consuming a lot of sweets can make your system a breeding ground for yeast infections. If you find that what you are eating is indeed contributing to yeast infection, eat more nuts, vegetables and fruits instead.

285.   Never sit in a wet bathing suit. Wet bathing suits mean a damp vaginal area, and this can cause a yeast infection. Be sure to dry off after swimming, and always change out of your suit as soon as you are able to. Staying dry is a great way to prevent those troublesome yeast infections.

286.   Always wipe from front to back. You probably don't give wiping much thought while you are in the

bathroom. Even so, it is important that you remember to wipe from front to back rather than back to front. The latter can spread harmful bacteria from your anus to your vagina.

287.   If you have to take antibiotics, be even more alert and proactive towards yeast infections. They're very helpful but can interfere with some of your natural bacteria. Healthy bacteria levels in your vagina are necessary to prevent yeast infections.

288.   A yeast infection in your mouth can be frightening. It often happens in infants, but can happen in adults as well. The best ways to fight an oral yeast infection is to rinse your mouth with warm salt water and avoid eating sugar. The salt water will flush out some yeast and not eating sugar will starve the yeast.

289.   Always use unscented products in your genital area. Each of these items can upset the natural chemical balance of a vagina, which then invites the risk of an infection. These products also stop you from smelling any odors that may signal the fact you have an infection.

290.   Reoccurring yeast infections are sometimes indicative of a serious medical problem. HIV, Leukemia and Diabetes can all cause problems with

the balance of flora in the vaginal area, and this can lead to a yeast infection. Visit your doctor if you have an ongoing problem with yeast infections to rule out any serious problems.

291.   When you are fighting off a yeast infection, avoid doing anything that weakens your immune system. This includes birth control pills and antibiotics. Douching also upsets the vaginal area locally, to a degree, that is not helpful. Give your body the chance to fight off the infection undisturbed by your actions.

292.   If you have recently been on antibiotics and suffered from a yeast infection following the treatment, you may have to talk with your doctor. You can get a preventative treatment from the doctor that will help reduce the chances of the yeast infection happening next time you take antibiotics for any reason.

293.   When you take acidophilus regularly, it can help you avoid yeast infections. The bacteria in these tablets promote a good balance of flora in your gut and the rest of your body. An imbalance inside your body is typically the culprit of most yeast infections.

294.   Avoid using scented products around your vagina. Using these can lead to yeast infections. If

you need something scented, apply perfume after you have showered and dressed.

295.   If you do not want a yeast infection, always wear a pair of cotton underwear underneath your pantyhose. Failing to do so creates a dark moist environment that is the perfect breeding ground for a yeast infection. Underwear that is cotton and white is best, as nylon and lycra do not breathe enough.

296.   The beneficial bacteria that is found in plain yogurt can be a natural yeast fighter. Yogurt can be applied topically, but some find it a bit messy and prefer to ingest it instead. It is essential that you purchase plain, unsweetened yogurt, because the sugars in sweetened yogurt can actually feed the yeast and cause it to flourish.

297.   If you notice that you are not getting enough sleep, make sure that you are getting at least eight hours per day. This can also be broken down into naps as the day wears on, as sleep will help to get your body back to the functional level to prevent infections all around.

298.   When your yeast infection is causing real pain, over-the-counter painkillers are a great treatment. Due to the impact the discomfort can have on your

day, you want to ensure that you are able to minimize the effects you are feeling as much as you can.

299.   One of the ways that you can prevent yeast infections altogether is to limit the alcohol intake that you consume during the day and night. Alcohol can hurt your immune system, which is a very important component in fighting the fungus that can lead to moderate and severe yeast infections.

300.   As much as you may enjoy taking hot baths, they could be causing your yeast infections. The organisms that cause yeast infections prefer warm and even hot environments. If you want to take a bath, try to take a warm one and do not stay in there for too long.

301.   Consume some live culture yogurt. Eat some yogurt to help your body get full of healthy bacteria in order to fight off yeast infections. Yogurt is filled with healthy bacteria called acidophilus cultures. This gives your body the healthy bacteria it needs to diminish the yeast.

302.   If you continue having yeast infections over and over again, it's time to visit your doctor. Using over-the-counter remedies is fine for most women. However, if you find your yeast infections keep

coming back, your doctor needs to check things out to make sure there is not some other underlying condition contributing to them.

303.   If you use an inhaler to treat your asthma, you should wash it at least once a week. Using a dirty inhaler can cause you to develop a yeast infection in your mouth and throat. If you have an infected mouth, wash your inhaler thoroughly every time you use it.

304.   Yeast infections can cause a discharge that can end up staining your underwear and causing it to develop an odor. You can help combat this problem by wearing a panty-liner in your underwear until your yeast infection has cleared up. This will help to keep your underpants stain free, and also help you to control the odor by changing the pads frequently.

305.   To relieve the burning and itching of a yeast infection, apply the juice from an aloe vera plant. You can also apply the juice to a cotton pad, place it in the fridge, and apply the cool liquid for soothing relief. Note that the aloe does not fight the yeast--it merely soothes the external symptoms.

306.   Seek out causes if you're a person that seems to constantly suffer from yeast infections. If you can't

quickly put your finger on the cause, think about your lifestyle habits. Clothing and diet are two huge factors in the formation of yeast infections, which you should look into.

307.   Many people are unaware that a poor diet can lead to increased frequency of yeast infections. Your body needs the proper fuel to keep it healthy, and if you are eating at the drive-thru every night, you are not getting the appropriate nutrition to keep your body healthy and fight off yeast infections.

308.   There are many natural remedies for yeast infections, but be careful not to overdo them. Many taught the benefits of vinegar, but too much vinegar will irritate the skin. Some say applying yogurt the vaginal area is a great cure, but yogurt contains sugar. Too much sugar will have a negative effect. Use natural remedies sparingly and only under the advice of your physician.

309.   If you have an infection around the area of your throat, it is likely that your saliva is harboring yeast. You should avoid putting things in your mouth and use plastic silverware and paper cups. Also, disinfect or purchase a new toothbrush to prevent recurring infection. You also need to avoid kissing anyone for a week after your infection has disappeared.

310.   Try to reduce your stress levels. Too much stress can weaken your immune system and leave you more susceptible to yeast infections. Try to avoid stress as a preventative measure. If you are currently suffering from a yeast infection, remaining too stressed out might exacerbate your infection. Practice some calming activities.

311.   Know the differences between yeast infections and bacterial infections. A yeast infection causes itching, burning, redness and discharge that looks like cottage cheese. Bacterial infections cause foul smells, itching, irritation and discharge that may appear yellowish or greenish in color. If you aren't sure which type you have, seek medical attention before attempting treatment.

312.   If you want to prevent yeast infections, you should try to incorporate yogurt into your diet. Live culture yogurt is the best for preventing yeast infections. The yogurt needs to be sugar free in order for it to be effective. If you do get a yeast infection, you can use sugar free yogurt as a topical cream as well.

313.   After you get out of the shower or bath, make sure that you dry off your body well, with a cotton towel. If you do not make sure to dry off well, you give the yeast somewhere to breed. Dry the best

you can and use a feminine powder if you need to be.

314.   After you come out of a pool, shed your wet clothing and dry off immediately. Do not spend any more time in damp clothing than you have to, because it creates an ideal environment for yeast growth. Also, don't forget to dry your vaginal area after taking off your wet clothes.

315.   The best way to prevent yeast infections is to dress properly. Cotton and silk are natural fibers that absorb moisture and will help keep the area dry. Nylon and other man made fabrics will not absorb moisture as well, and you will increase the likelihood of getting a yeast infection.

316.   The organisms that cause yeast infections love warmth and moist areas of the body. Try to limit your exposure in hot tubs and long hot baths. Doing this will reduce the chances of you getting a yeast infection. In the summer, try not to wear clothing that is too tight that will trap hot air around the vagina.

317.   Do not douche. The notion that douching cleanses the vagina is a misconception, as it actually cleanses itself. Douching removes the beneficial strains of bacteria that help to keep yeast under

control, too. This can lead to even more frequent or severe yeast infections. If you experience persistent discomfort or a bad smell, see your doctor--you may have a more serious infection.

318.   Keep your vaginal area dry and clean. Yeast infections are more likely to occur if you do not. Be sure to wash regularly. Wear absorbent panties, like cotton. This will help to keep your vaginal area dry throughout the day, thus decreasing the likelihood of you developing a yeast infection.

319.   In order to prevent yeast infections, good hygiene is key. Thoroughly clean the vaginal area getting between all of the folds of the skin. Next, dry your genital area thoroughly; you may even want to think about using a hair dryer in order to get this task done effectively. Yeast will grow in moist areas, so being as dry as possible can really help.

320.   If you are suffering from a yeast infection and sexually active, you might need to cut out sex for a little while. Sex can transmit yeast infections from one partner to the other, and the activity can also make your yeast infection worse. Stop the act until you are able to receive a full treatment and cure your infection.

321.   Clean cotton underwear is something you should wear to stop yeast infections from occurring. Natural fibers like cotton are less likely to irritate your skin and are better able to deal with moisture. When you have recurring infections, consider what your underwear are made of. If moisture is a problem, use feminine napkins.

322.   There are many natural remedies for yeast infections, but be careful not to overdo them. Many taught the benefits of vinegar, but too much vinegar will irritate the skin. Some say applying yogurt the vaginal area is a great cure, but yogurt contains sugar. Too much sugar will have a negative effect. Use natural remedies sparingly and only under the advice of your physician.

323.   Although it may seem counterintuitive, avoid vaginal wash to prevent yeast infections. Vaginal wash products are often scented and can be irritating. Using these on an ongoing basis can upset the natural balance of the good bacteria in your body. Sometimes chronic vaginal wash use can even completely destroy your healthy natural bacteria.

324.   Try to keep your stress under control. It has not been proven in scientific studies, but many people have observed that stress is linked to yeast infections. If you are often stressed out or have a

highly stressful job, try to manage your stress the best you can by using meditation, yoga, or deep breathing.

325.   Taking antibiotics for a long period of time can cause you to develop yeast infections. If this happens to you, you should immediately stop taking your antibiotics and contact your doctor. If you have developed yeast infections during the past because of antibiotics, you should let your doctor know about it before he or she prescribes you antibiotics.

326.   When you use the restroom, do not wipe from back to front. If you do, you could be spreading bacteria from your anus to your vagina. The bacteria could lead to serious yeast infections and other vaginal infections. Always wipe yourself from front to back with soft, dry toilet paper.

327.   In order to fight yeast infections, consider making some changes in your diet. Several studies have shown that simple sugars can promote yeast infections, while live culture yogurts can help to diminish yeast infections.

328.   Keep your water intake high. You should drink between 8-10 glasses of water every day, but you should drink even more when fighting an infection.

Drinking more causes you to urinate more. This lets you get out extra sugar which yeast likes to eat.

329.   If you do not want a yeast infection, always wear a pair of cotton underwear underneath your pantyhose. Failing to do so creates a dark moist environment that is the perfect breeding ground for a yeast infection. Underwear that is cotton and white is best, as nylon and lycra do not breathe enough.

330.   If you find yourself suffering from chronic yeast infections, you might need to avoid foods that are high in yeast and mold. If your body is already having a difficult time warding off yeast, you don't want to aggravate that condition by consuming more yeast and mold. Foods to avoid would include things like dried fruits, melons, peanuts and most cheeses.

www.ingramcontent.com/pod-product-compliance
Lightning Source LLC
Chambersburg PA
CBHW060747260726
48660CB00002B/517